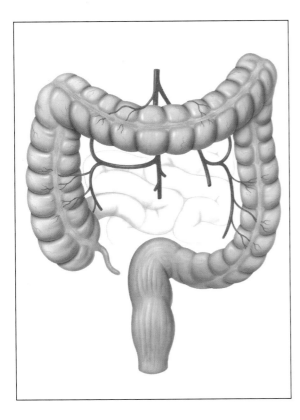

THE STOMACH

AND

DIGESTIVE

SYSTEM

Carol Ballard

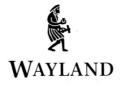

WAYLAND

TITLES IN THE SERIES

The Heart and Circulatory System
The Stomach and Digestive System
The Brain and Nervous System
The Lungs and Respiratory System
The Skeleton and Muscular System
The Reproductive System

Editor: Ruth Raudsepp
Medical illustrator: Michael Courtney
Series designer: Rita Storey
Production controller: Carol Titchener
Consultant: Dr. Tony Smith, Associate Editor of the British Medical Journal

First published in 1996 by Wayland Publishers Limited
61 Western Road, Hove, East Sussex BN3 1JD, England.

British Library Cataloguing in Publication Data
Ballard, Carol
The Stomach and Digestive System (The human body series)
1. Stomach - Juvenile literature 2. Digestive organs - Juvenile literature
I. Title
612. 3
ISBN 0-7502-1765-0

Picture Acknowledgements
The publishers would like to thank the following for use of their photographs:
National Medical Slide Bank 8, 28; Science Photo Library 19, 23, 25, 26, 29,
35, 43; The remaining pictures are from the Wayland Picture Library.

Typeset by Storey Books
Printed and bound by L.E.G.O. S.p A., Vicenza, Italy.

CONTENTS

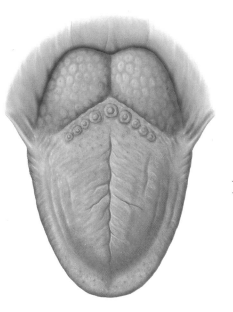

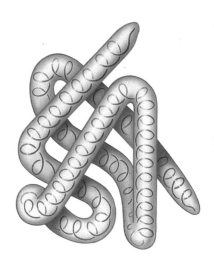

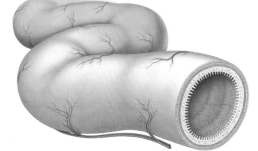

Introduction

The body uses food and liquids for energy, growth, maintenance and repair. Before it can do this, the food has to be broken down into smaller and simpler pieces. This 'breaking down' process is called **digestion**. It is carried out by the digestive system. The digestive system is really just one long tube. Digestion begins in the mouth, when food is chewed. Then, food is gradually broken down into separate chemicals as it travels down the tube. The parts of food that the body can use are collected by the blood, and the waste material that is left leaves the body when you go to the toilet.

Digestion begins in the mouth. Find out more on page 6.

The stomach contains chemicals to digest food. Find out more on page 18.

Food is absorbed from the small intestine by the blood. Find out more on page 24.

Water is taken out of the waste material by the large intestine. Find out more on page 26.

The liver is like a large chemical factory. Find out more on page 30.

It is important to eat a balanced diet to make sure that the body gets all the different types of food it needs. Find out more on page 36.

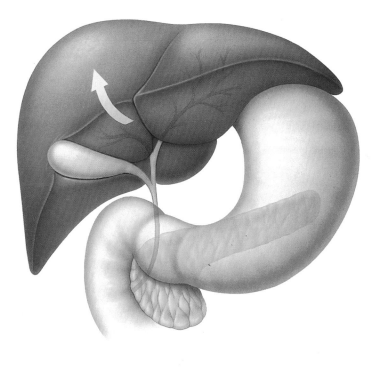

◀ **The liver, stomach, gall bladder and pancreas. Organs involved in the digestion of food.**

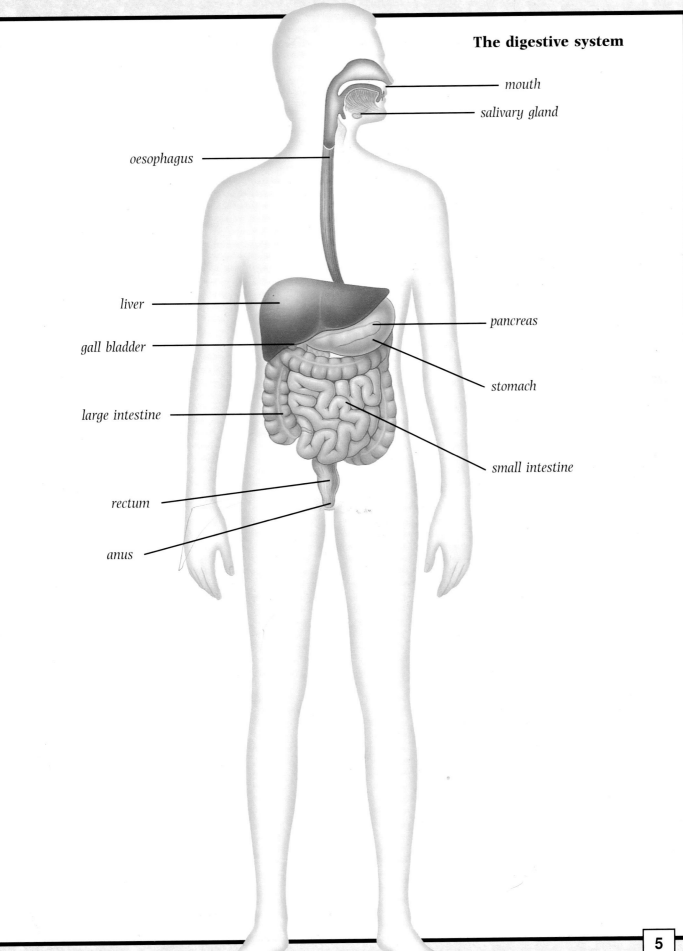

mouth

salivary gland

oesophagus

liver

pancreas

gall bladder

stomach

large intestine

small intestine

rectum

anus

In the mouth

When a bite of food is taken, the mouth begins the process of digestion.

The teeth are used for chewing food. They make it softer and break it into smaller and smaller pieces. Chewing is usually an automatic reflex action – we do it without thinking about it. It is triggered by the feel of food against the teeth and the inside of the mouth. As the jaw muscles relax, the jaw drops. Other muscles pull the jaw back up again. This action crushes the food between the back teeth. Muscles also move the jaw from side to side, grinding the food between the teeth. During chewing, a liquid called **saliva** is produced by glands around and under the tongue. Saliva helps to lubricate the food, making it easy to swallow. It also contains chemicals that begin to digest the food. The tongue moves food around the mouth, helping to make sure it is mixed with saliva. As food touches the tongue, its taste is detected. The nose detects the smell of the food, which helps to make the flavour clearer and stronger.

Food eaten is often much colder than the body (like ice-cream) or much hotter than the body (like pizza). If very hot or very cold food is swallowed it can be uncomfortable and even damage the foodpipe. While food is in the mouth, it is warmed or cooled until it is nearer body temperature, making it comfortable and safe to swallow. When food is swallowed, a flap called the epiglottis blocks off the entrance to the windpipe so that food cannot 'go down the wrong way'. The soft palate rises to stop food entering the nasal cavity.

FACT BOX

Babies are born without teeth. Their first teeth emerge at about six months.

Children have twenty milk teeth.
Adults have thirty-two permanent teeth.

Teeth come in many shapes and sizes. Each type of tooth helps to break up the food that is eaten.

All the different foods tasted on the tongue are combinations of sweet, sour, salty and bitter.

**Cross-section of the mouth ▶
showing the structures
involved in chewing and
swallowing.**

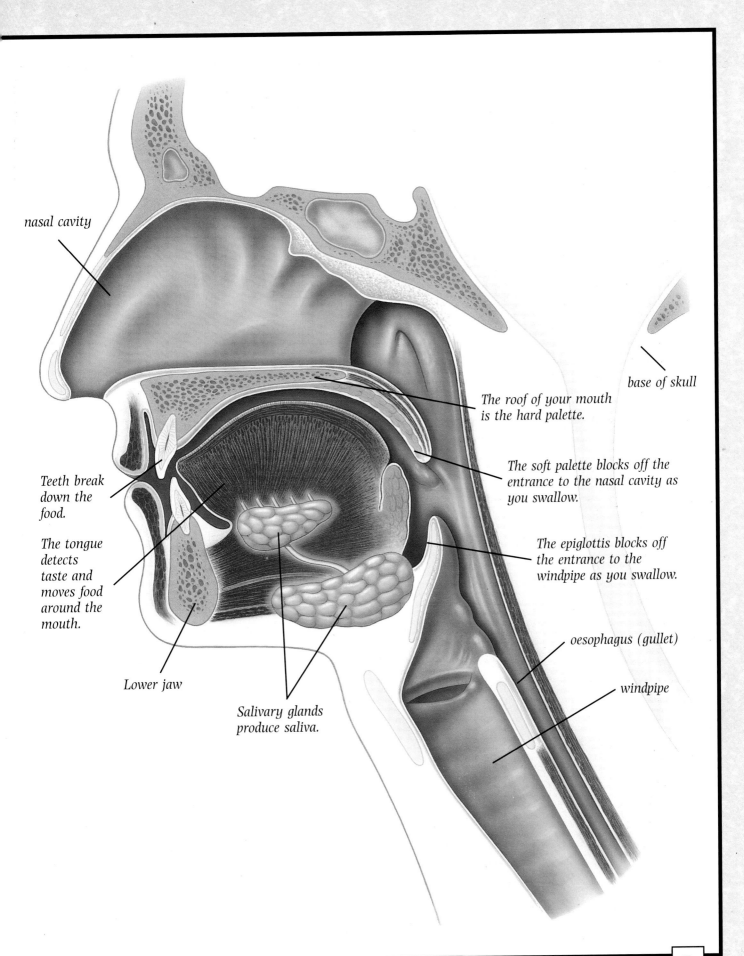

nasal cavity

base of skull

The roof of your mouth is the hard palette.

The soft palette blocks off the entrance to the nasal cavity as you swallow.

Teeth break down the food.

The tongue detects taste and moves food around the mouth.

The epiglottis blocks off the entrance to the windpipe as you swallow.

oesophagus (gullet)

windpipe

Lower jaw

Salivary glands produce saliva.

Teeth

Babies are born without teeth. After about six months of age, the first set of twenty teeth, called the milk teeth, start to push their way through the gums. At about six years of age, the permanent teeth begin to push through the gums. They loosen the milk teeth that are in their way and the milk teeth fall out. At about twelve years of age, most people have twenty-eight of their permanent set of thirty-two teeth. The remaining four teeth, the back molars, or wisdom teeth, rarely appear before the age of seventeen, and sometimes they do not appear at all.

Different types of teeth have different jobs to do. At the front of the mouth are flat, sharp teeth called incisors. These are good at nibbling food.

Adults have eight incisor teeth, four in the upper jaw and four in the lower jaw. At the sides of the mouth are sharp, pointed teeth called canines. These are good at ripping and tearing food. There are four canine teeth in an adult's mouth, one at each side of the upper and lower incisor teeth. At the back of the mouth are strong, flat teeth. The first one on each side is called a premolar and the back three on each side are called molars. These have a large, knobbly surface and are good for grinding and crushing food.

Many animals eat only one kind of food, so they need one type of tooth. We eat a wide range of foods and so need different types of teeth to enable us to bite, snip, grind and chew.

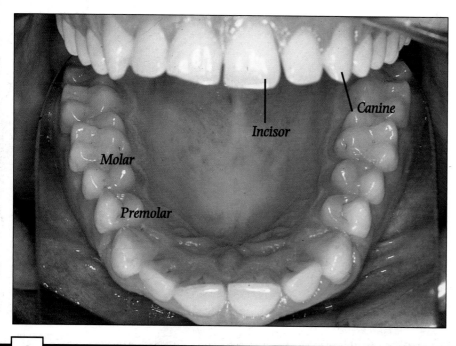

Incisor

Canine

Molar

Premolar

Adults have several different types of teeth, which are used for different jobs.

Only about half of each tooth can be seen because the other half is buried inside the gums. The part that is seen is called the crown and the part that is hidden by the gums is called the root.

Each tooth has several layers. The outside of a tooth is made of enamel. This is a thin, shiny layer, giving a hard surface for grinding and cutting. Enamel is made mainly of calcium and phosphorus, and is not a living layer. Below the enamel is a very hard layer called dentine. This is similar to bone, and is kept alive by the blood vessels in the centre, the pulp, which supply it with **nutrients** and oxygen. The pulp is a soft, living core. Nerves and blood vessels run though the pulp. The teeth are held in place in the jawbone by a layer of cement. This contains fibres that cushion the teeth and protect them.

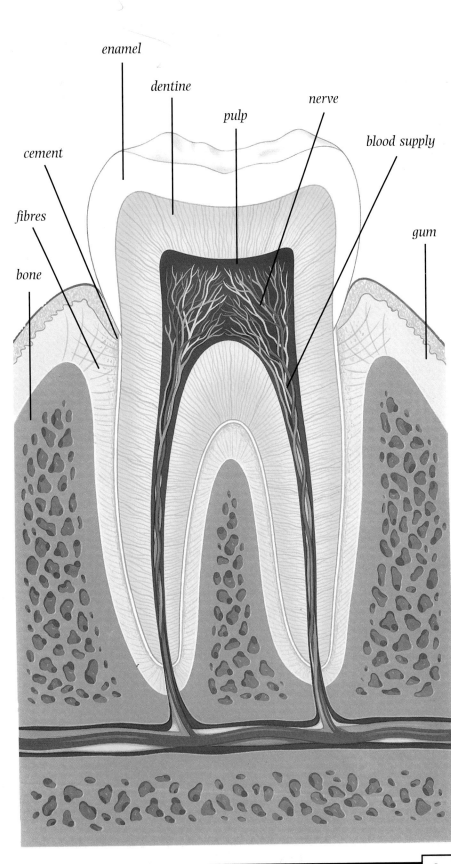

Cross-section through a molar showing enamel, dentine and pulp.

Look after your teeth

Teeth will only stay healthy and strong if they are looked after. Without care, they will develop tooth decay.

After a meal, tiny pieces of food may be left on the teeth. Bacteria in the mouth feed on the sugar in these tiny pieces of food, producing acid. This acid starts to eat into the teeth. Saliva is alkaline, and after an hour or so will neutralize the acid, but it is often too late – the damage may already be done. The hole in the tooth made by the acid is called a cavity. The tiny cavity made by the acid eating through the enamel layer would not cause any pain and so would go unnoticed. But as the acid gradually begins to damage the dentine below, mild toothache may be felt. The acid may eat right through the dentine layer and into the pulp, which is very painful. Bacteria begin to infect the cavity that has formed. The infection may spread through the pulp, killing it and forming an abscess, which is extremely painful. To remove the decayed parts of a tooth and stop further decay, the dentist uses a drill. The hole is filled with material like putty. It dries very quickly to form a hard surface to bite on.

If teeth are not cleaned regularly, a layer of bacteria can build up on the teeth. This is called **plaque**. If not removed, plaque can spread between the gum and the enamel of the teeth and cause an infection called gingivitis. The gums look very red and may start to bleed. If allowed to get worse, the gums shrink a little and the teeth become loose and eventually fall out. Plaque can also become very hard, forming a layer called tartar. Dentists can only remove this by chipping it off.

FACT BOX

Brush the teeth regularly, morning and night. A toothbrush will remove bacteria and bits of food from the surface of the teeth. Dental floss is good for cleaning between teeth. Disclosing tablets stain plaque bright red so that following brushing you can check that all the plaque has been removed.

Finish a meal with a hard vegetable, such as a raw carrot, and rinse the mouth with water.

Try not to eat sweets or drink sugary drinks between meals.

Visit the dentist every six months.

1. Tiny scraps of food are left on the teeth. Bacteria feed on this and produce acid. The acid begins to eat into the enamel, making a small hole (cavity).

▼

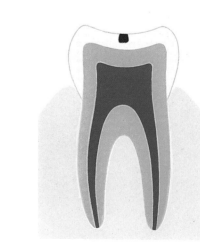

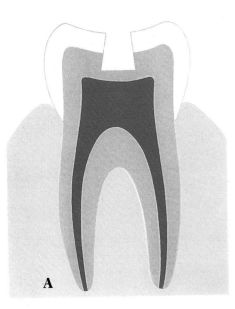

A

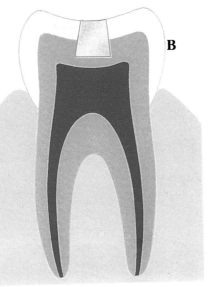

B

◀ A. The dentist uses a drill to remove the decayed parts of the tooth.

B. The hole is filled up with a putty-like material. It dries very quickly to form a hard surface to bite on.

2. As the acid eats further into the tooth, the cavity gets bigger.

▼

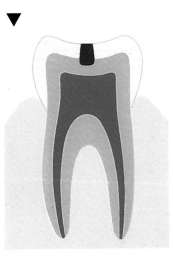

3. The cavity reaches the pulp. The nerve is exposed and severe toothache is felt.

▼

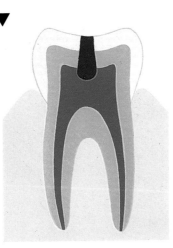

4. Germs reach the base of the tooth, forming an abscess that causes extreme pain.

▼

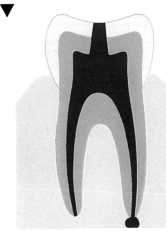

Tasting food

Both the mouth and nose play an important part in allowing us to taste the many different flavours of foods and drinks.

The tongue has special cells that detect different tastes. These cells are clustered together in small groups called taste buds. Only four types of taste can be distinguished by the taste buds: sweet, sour, salty and bitter. Each taste bud can only detect one of these tastes. All the taste buds which detect one taste are in one area of the tongue, so different types of taste are detected by different parts of the tongue. The tip of the tongue detects salty and sweet tastes. The sides of the tongue detect sour tastes and the back of the tongue detects bitter tastes. The taste buds respond to chemicals in food by sending electrical signals along the nerves to the brain. The brain knows which taste buds have sent the signals, so it can work out exactly what it is you are tasting.

The upper lining of the nose has special sensitive cells that can detect smells. Chemicals in the air brush over tiny bristly hairs, which stimulate the sensitive cells to send electrical signals along the nerves to the brain. The brain works out which chemicals have been detected and adds the information to the signals received from the taste buds. Then the brain translates all the information and sends a message about the flavour of the food. The sensitive cells in the nose can detect many more chemicals than the taste buds. This is why, when you have a cold and your nose is blocked, your food may not seem to taste quite the same as usual.

The position of the taste buds on the tongue. ▼

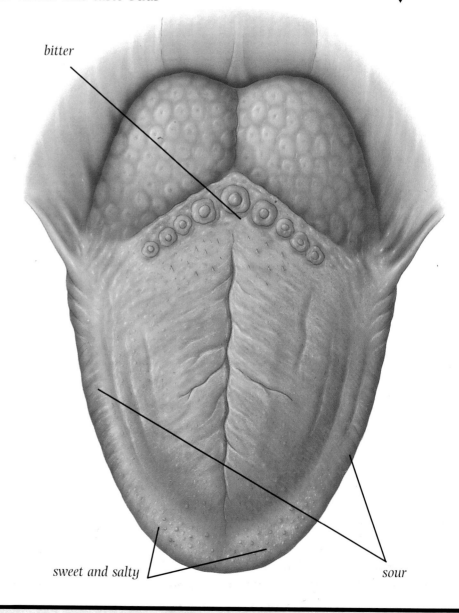

bitter

sweet and salty

sour

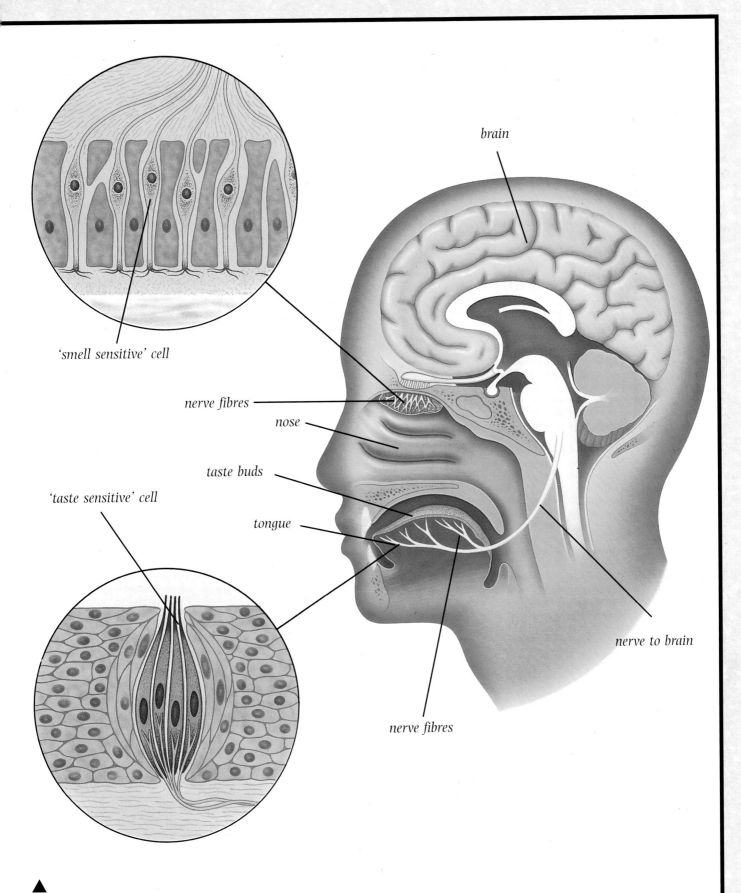

'smell sensitive' cell

nerve fibres

nose

taste buds

'taste sensitive' cell

tongue

brain

nerve to brain

nerve fibres

▲
**Cross-section of the side view of the head showing the
position of taste buds and smell receptors.**

Food digestion in the mouth

Digestion of food begins with chewing. The teeth crush and grind the food into smaller and smaller pieces. As food is chewed, it is mixed with saliva. This helps to soften and lubricate the food, making it easier to swallow. Saliva also contains special chemicals called **enzymes** which begin to break the food down. The enzymes in saliva are amylase enzymes, which attack starch molecules. The enzymes act like 'chemical scissors', chopping the very long starch molecules into smaller pieces.

When the food is soft enough, the tongue pushes upwards and backwards, moulding the food into a round lump called a bolus. The tongue pushes the bolus of food to the back of the mouth. At the back of the mouth, the pressure of the bolus forces the soft palate upwards. This blocks off the nasal cavity, stopping food entering. The epiglottis blocks the entrance to the windpipe to stop food entering. When we swallow, the bolus of food is pushed

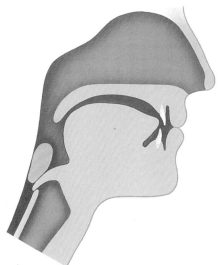

1. A bolus of food is pushed to the back of the mouth.

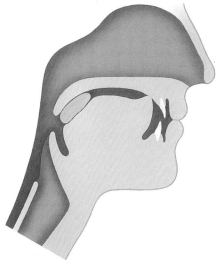

2. The soft palate blocks the nasal cavity.

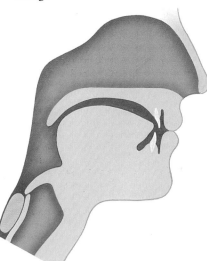

3. The epiglottis blocks the windpipe.

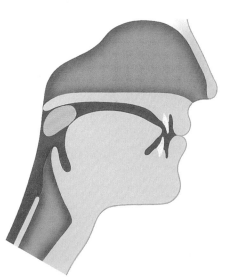

4. The bolus of food is pushed into the oesophagus.

The process of swallowing.

out of the mouth and into the oesophagus. We can control the beginning actions of swallowing, these are voluntary actions. But when food touches the back of the mouth, the actions become automatic and cannot be controlled, These are involuntary or reflex actions.

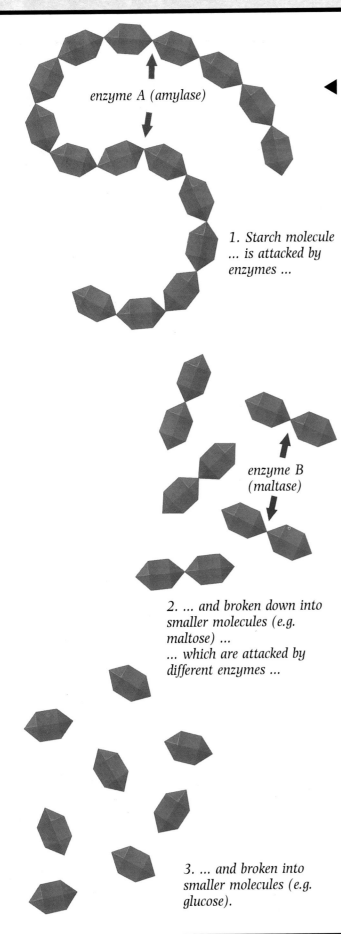

enzyme A (amylase)

◀ **Long starch molecules are chopped into smaller molecules by amylase enzymes in saliva.**

*1. Starch molecule
... is attacked by
enzymes ...*

*enzyme B
(maltase)*

*2. ... and broken down into
smaller molecules (e.g.
maltose) ...
... which are attacked by
different enzymes ...*

*3. ... and broken into
smaller molecules (e.g.
glucose).*

FACT BOX

It takes between twelve and thirty-six hours for a meal to pass through the digestive system.

Nearly 2 litres of saliva are produced by the salivary glands every day.

An adult's digestive system is about 9 metres long.

The surface of the small intestine is folded so tightly that it has a surface area of about 20 square metres.

The oesophagus

The oesophagus lies just behind the windpipe. It connects the mouth to the stomach. In an adult, the oesophagus is about 25 cm long. The walls of the oesophagus are made up of several layers. The outer layer is the serosa. This is a thin layer of connective tissue. Underneath the serosa is a layer of muscles. These are longitudinal muscles and they run along the length of the oesophagus. Underneath the outer muscle layer is another layer of muscles. These are circular muscles and they run in rings around the oesophagus. The submucosa lies underneath the circular muscles. This is a tough, elastic layer and contains blood vessels and nerves. The inner layer of the oesophagus is the mucosa. This layer is coated with a slimy liquid called mucus. Although different parts are specialized in different ways, the whole of the digestive system has a similar, basic layered structure.

Food cannot move along the oesophagus by itself, it has to be pushed. The muscles in the walls of the oesophagus contract and relax in turn to push the food along. The ring of muscle behind the food bolus contracts, and at the same time the ring of muscle in front of the bolus relaxes. The bolus is squeezed forward into the space where the muscles are relaxed. These muscles then contract in turn, and the next ring of muscle relaxes, so the bolus is squeezed forward again. The outer longitudinal muscles also contract and relax. As they contract, a portion of the oesophagus is shortened, pushing the bolus forward.

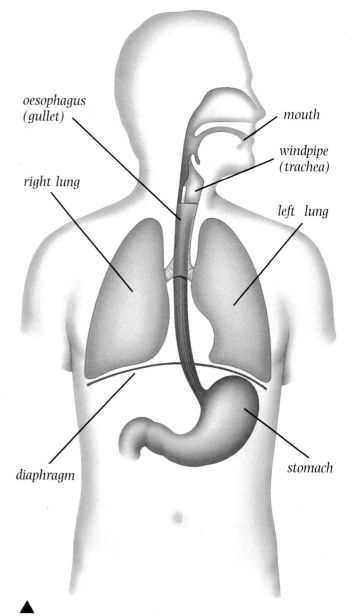

oesophagus (gullet)

mouth

windpipe (trachea)

right lung

left lung

diaphragm

stomach

▲ This diagram shows the position of the oesophagus in the upper body.

This diagram shows the inside of the ▶ oesophagus.

The contraction and relaxation of the muscles move along the oesophagus like a wave. This process is called **peristalsis**, and the wave-like motion is called a peristaltic wave. Food is moved through the whole of the digestive system by a series of peristaltic waves, moving more quickly in some parts than others. The peristaltic waves in the oesophagus travel at about 4 cm per second, so food can travel from your mouth to your stomach in about 5 or 6 seconds.

At the bottom of the oesophagus is a ring of muscle called the oesophageal sphincter. This is usually tightly shut, but when food arrives the muscles relax to allow food to enter the stomach. The muscles then contract again, closing the entrance to the stomach. Sometimes, the oesophageal sphincter does not close properly. This causes a burning sensation (heartburn), as the acidic stomach contents move up into the bottom of the oesophagus. The oesophageal sphincter may not close properly when the abdominal muscles contract during breathing, or during the late stages of pregnancy.

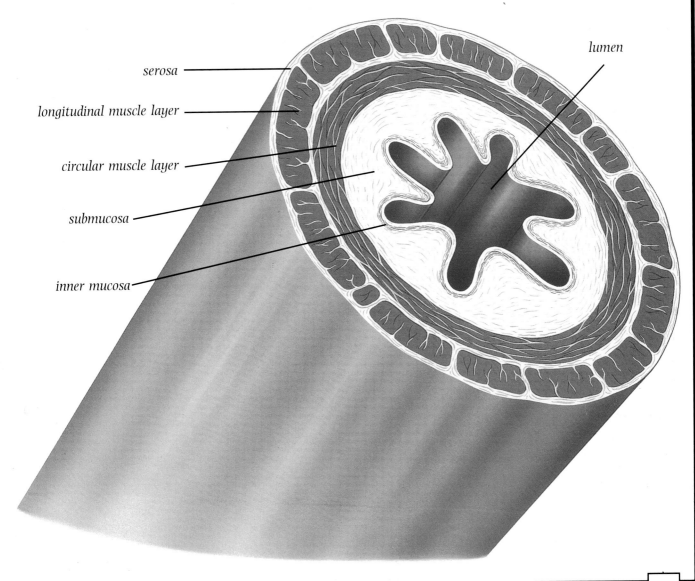

serosa

longitudinal muscle layer

circular muscle layer

submucosa

inner mucosa

lumen

The stomach

An adult's stomach is about 25 cm long. It is a J-shaped bag with strong, muscular walls which can stretch to allow the stomach to hold a meal.

There are three areas of the stomach: the upper part is the fundus, the middle part is called the body and the lower part is the pylorus. Long muscles run along the length of the stomach and circular bands of muscle go round it. These muscles contract and relax about three times every minute, churning the food up and making sure it is mixed very thoroughly with **gastric** juices. The stomach is made up of the same layers as the oesophagus: the serosa, muscles, submucosa and mucosa. The mucosa contains gastric glands which produce a liquid called gastric juice. This contains hydrochloric acid, which acts on protein molecules in food by unraveling them. This makes it easier for enzymes to work. It also kills bacteria in the food, helping to keep the digestive system free from infection. Gastric juice also contains

pepsin, an enzyme which breaks long protein molecules into smaller molecules (polypeptides). The lining of the stomach is protected by a layer of mucus, preventing the gastric juices from damaging the stomach itself.

Different foods stay in the stomach for different lengths of time. Starches and sugars stay for one or two hours, proteins stay for three to five hours and fats may stay even longer.

The action of the gastric juice and the churning by the stomach muscles eventually turn the food into a liquid. This liquid food is called **chyme.** It moves out of the stomach through a ring of muscle called the pyloric sphincter. This is usually tightly shut, to prevent the stomach contents leaving the stomach before they are ready. When it opens, a wave of contraction pushes some of the food out of the stomach and into the small intestine.

The parts of the stomach.
▼

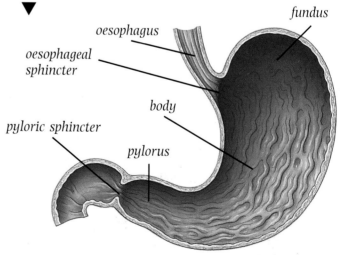

bands of muscle

oesophagus

oesophageal sphincter

fundus

body

pyloric sphincter

pylorus

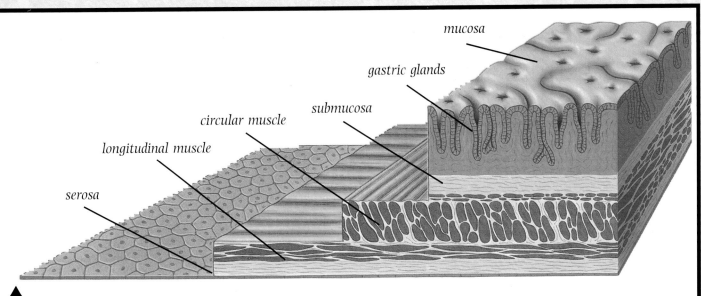

mucosa

gastric glands

submucosa

circular muscle

longitudinal muscle

serosa

▲

A cross-section through the stomach wall showing muscles and gastric glands that produce gastric juice.

A patient may be given a 'barium meal', a liquid that allows doctors to see the structure of the digestive system on an X-ray. Doctors also use a flexible instrument called an endoscope to view the digestive system. The endoscope is swallowed and pictures are transmitted back to a screen. ▶

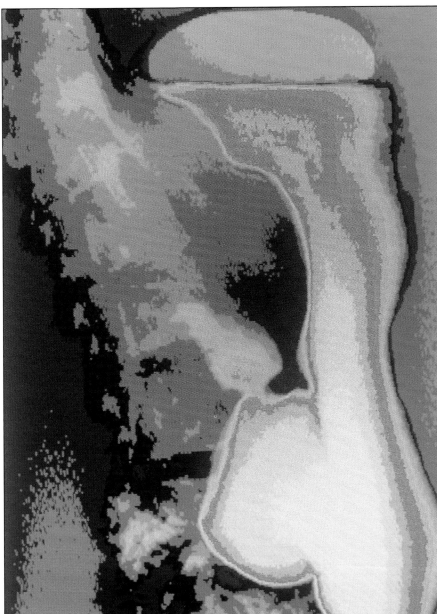

If there is something wrong with the food you have eaten, you may vomit. Waves of contraction push the food in the opposite direction. It is forced violently out of the stomach, up the oesophagus and out through the mouth. This defence mechanism allows the body to reject poisons and harmful substances.

The duodenum

When the liquid food (chyme) leaves the stomach via the pyloric sphincter, it enters the first part of the small intestine, the duodenum.

This is curved round into a horseshoe shape and is about 20 cm long. Like the rest of the digestive system, it is made up of several layers.

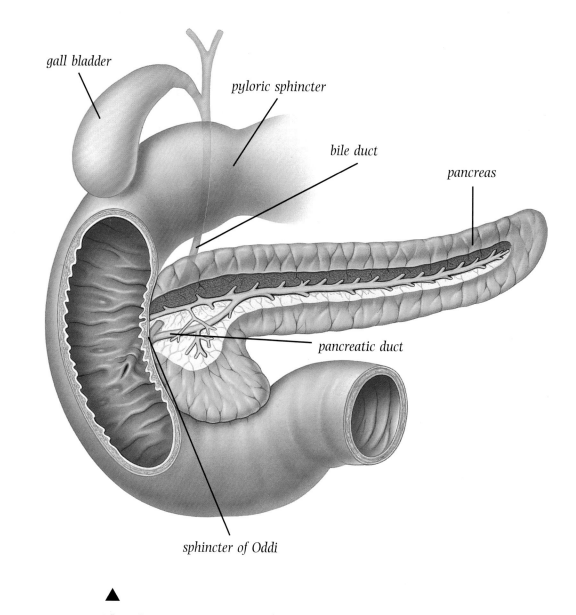

gall bladder

pyloric sphincter

bile duct

pancreas

pancreatic duct

sphincter of Oddi

▲

This diagram shows the duodenum and the position of the pancreas and gall bladder around it.

The layers of longitudinal and circular muscle in the duodenum contract and relax regularly, so food is moved along by peristaltic waves. The mucosa of the duodenum contains glands which produce digestive juices. When chyme enters the duodenum it is very acidic. If it continued to travel through the digestive system, the acid would cause a lot of damage. Chemicals produced in the duodenum help to neutralize the acid, making it safe for the chyme to continue moving through the digestive system.

The stomach enzyme, pepsin, can only work in an acid environment, so the alkaline environment of the duodenum stops it breaking down proteins. Instead, glands in the duodenal wall produce enzymes called peptidases, which finish the digestion of proteins by chopping up polypeptides into much smaller molecules (**amino acids**). Maltase and sucrase are enzymes also produced by glands in the duodenal wall. These enzymes turn maltose and sucrose (types of sugar that the body cannot use) into **glucose**, which it can use.

In the duodenum, digestive juices from the liver and pancreas are mixed with the liquid food. They enter the duodenum through a small hole in the duodenal wall. This is controlled by a ring of muscle called the sphincter of Oddi. **Bile**, which is made in the liver and stored in the gall bladder, plays an important role in the digestion of fats. Pancreatic juice enters the duodenum and contains enzymes to break down proteins, starch and fats.

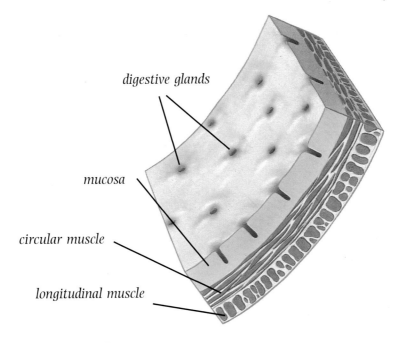

digestive glands

mucosa

circular muscle

longitudinal muscle

▲

This diagram shows what the duodenum and pancreas look like inside.

The pancreas and gall bladder

The pancreas is a small organ, about 15 cm long and lies just behind the stomach. It has two functions:

1. It produces pancreatic juice which it releases into the duodenum.
2. It produces a hormone called **insulin** which it releases into the bloodstream.

Pancreatic juice contains several enzymes which carry on the process of digestion. These enzymes are made by special cells (acinar cells) which are grouped together in clusters like bunches of grapes. The pancreatic juice is collected in a network of tiny tubes. These join up with each other and eventually form a large tube called the pancreatic duct. Pancreatic juice leaves the pancreas via the pancreatic duct and enters the duodenum. The enzymes in pancreatic juice are very strong. To stop them damaging the pancreas itself, they are produced in an 'inactive' form. They become active when they reach the alkaline contents of the duodenum. The enzymes in pancreatic juice include: trypsin and chymotrypsin which break down proteins into smaller molecules; amylase, which splits starch and changes it into maltose; and lipase, which begins to digest fats, changing them into **fatty acids** and glycerol.

Insulin is produced by small groups of cells in the pancreas called islets of Langerhans. They take their name from Paul Langerhans, a nineteenth-century German pathologist who discovered them. Insulin is released straight into the bloodstream and taken to the liver. It plays an important part in controlling how much sugar is in the blood.

The gall bladder is a muscular bag about 8 cm long which is tucked behind the lobes of the liver. It stores a green, watery liquid called bile which is made in the liver. As food moves along the duodenum, the muscles of the gall bladder contract, forcing bile out into the bile duct. The bile travels along the bile duct, which eventually joins the pancreatic duct. Bile enters the duodenum, and mixes with the food. Bile does not contain enzymes, but chemicals called bile salts, which attack fats in food, breaking them down into smaller pieces. These small droplets of fat are then attacked by the enzyme, lipase, which breaks down fats even further.

Insulin is made by groups of cells called islets of Langerhans. These are surrounded by acinar cells which make digestive enzymes. ▶

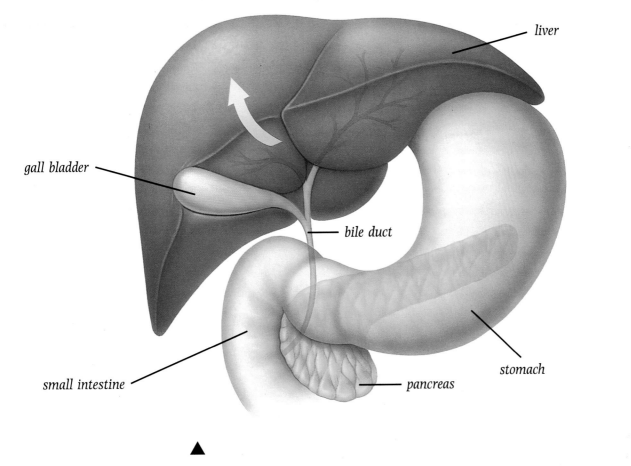

liver

gall bladder

bile duct

small intestine

pancreas

stomach

▲

The gall bladder is tucked behind the lobes of the liver.

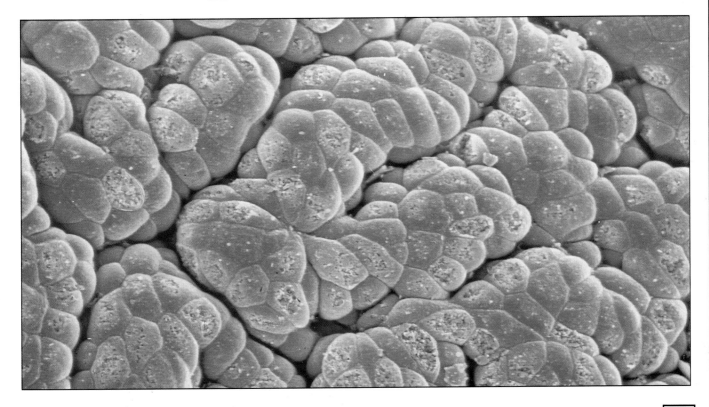

The small intestine

Food moves through the duodenum to the small intestine. This is a long, narrow tube, and although it is between 4 and 6 m long, it is coiled and looped tightly so that it fits into the abdominal space.

By the time the food reaches the small intestine, most of it is broken down into the separate units or molecules which the body can use. The process of digestion is more or less finished, but the nutrients have to get out of the digestive system and into the rest of the body. This process is called absorption, and it takes place as the digested food passes through the small intestine.

The small intestine is made up of several layers, like the rest of the digestive system. It has a rich blood supply, both to nourish the small intestine and to carry away the nutrients which are absorbed by the small intestine. The inner lining of the small intestine is specially

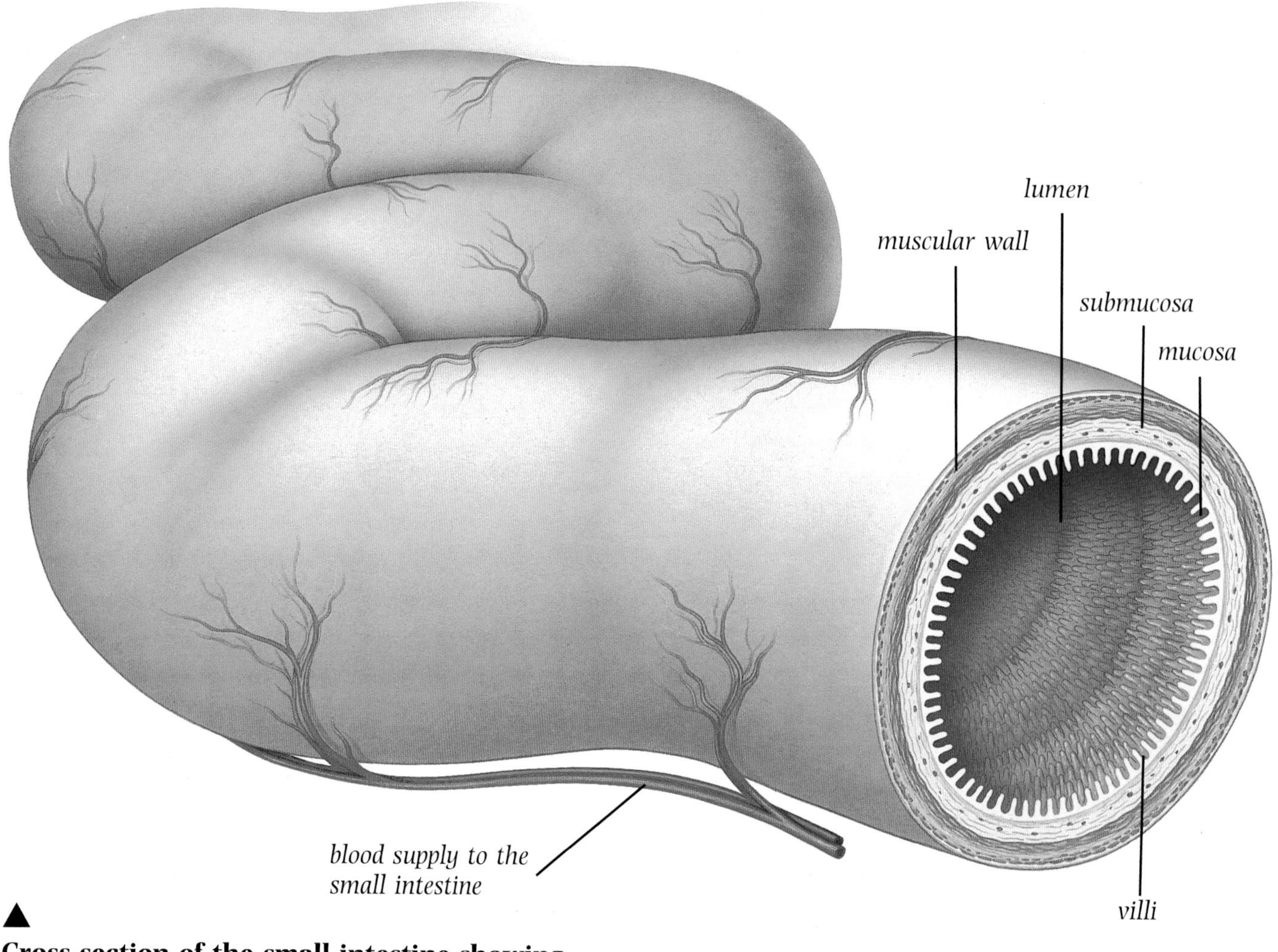

lumen

muscular wall

submucosa

mucosa

blood supply to the small intestine

villi

▲
Cross-section of the small intestine showing the villi and blood supply. Finger-like villi line the inside of the small intestine, creating an enormous surface area for the absorption of nutrients.

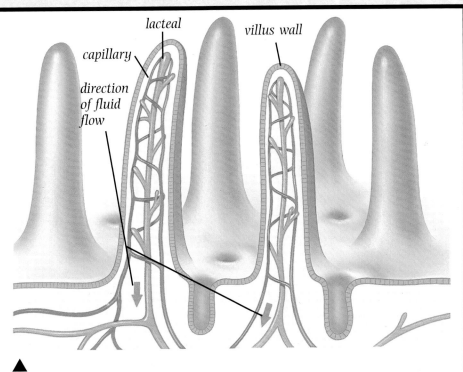

lacteal

capillary

villus wall

direction of fluid flow

▲
Each villus has its own blood capillary and lacteal.

adapted to make sure that nutrients are absorbed efficiently. It has millions of tiny finger-like structures called villi which point in towards the centre of the tube. Each villus is covered with even tinier 'fingers' called microvilli. These structures increase the surface area of the inside of the small intestine. Its surface area is about 600 times greater than it would be if it had a flat lining. Each villus has its own blood **capillary** and **lymph** vessel (**lacteal**). The nutrient molecules are small enough to pass through the walls of a villus. Amino acids (from proteins) and sugars pass from the villus into the blood capillary, and are carried away in the bloodstream. Fatty acids (from fats) pass into the lacteal and are carried away into the lymphatic system. Eventually they will also reach the blood stream.

The walls of the small intestine produce intestinal juice. This contains some digestive enzymes, but it is mainly mucus. It acts rather like oil, protecting and lubricating the inner lining of the small intestine so food can move along it smoothly.

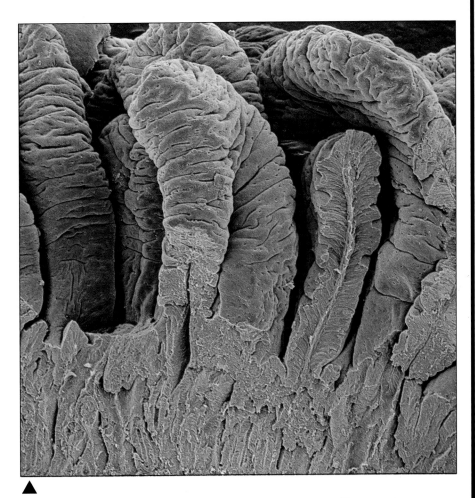

▲
Individual villi push into the centre of the small intestine.

The large intestine

The large intestine is also known as the colon. It is much shorter and fatter than the small intestine – about 1 m long and 6 cm in diameter. The first small section is the caecum. There are three main sections that follow the caecum: the ascending colon, the transverse colon and the descending colon. These three sections are like three sides of a square. The last part of the large intestine is the rectum. The appendix is a small structure that is attached to the large intestine. It does not play a part in the digestion or absorption of food, but it may be involved in the immune system.

All the useful material in food is absorbed before it reaches the large intestine. Only waste material and water, containing dissolved mineral salts, is left. The main function of the large intestine is to remove the water and salts from the waste. Food enters the large intestine through a valve called the ileocaecal sphincter. As it travels along the large intestine, water and mineral salts pass through the walls of the intestine. The water and minerals salts then enter blood capillaries and are carried away to be used by the body. Once the water is removed, the waste material becomes more solid, eventually forming the brown waste material called **faeces**. Faeces are stored in the rectum until they can be removed from the body when we go to the toilet. Faeces leave the body through another muscular valve called the anus. Unlike other valves in the digestive system, you can usually control the opening and closing of the anus. Even if you are

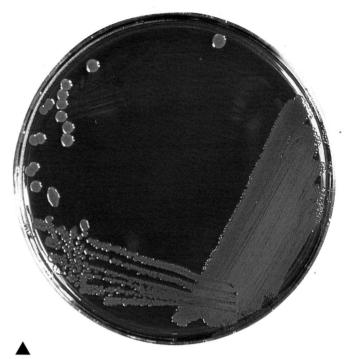

▲
This picture shows E-coli bacteria growing on a petri dish. E-coli bacteria normally live in the gut where they cause neither disease nor infection. However, if they find their way into the bladder they can cause a urinary infection. A simple step to prevent bacteria from being transferred to other sites in the body is to wash your hands thoroughly after going to the toilet.

perfectly healthy, your faeces may contain bacteria which can cause disease. You can avoid spreading diseases by following simple hygiene precautions such as washing your hands after going to the toilet.

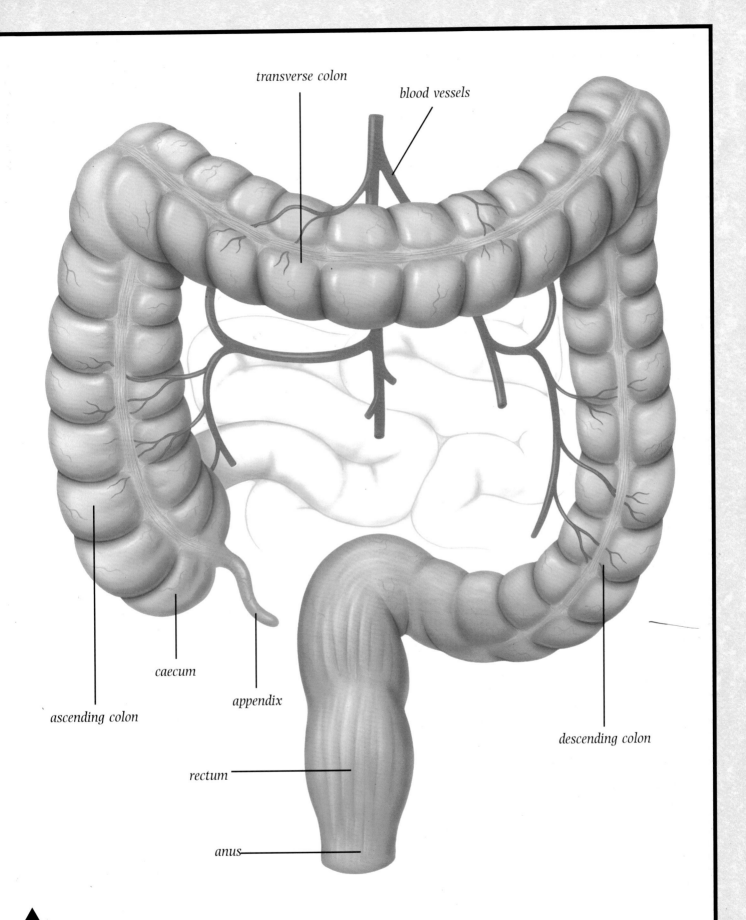

transverse colon

blood vessels

caecum

appendix

ascending colon

descending colon

rectum

anus

▲
This diagram shows the parts of the large intestine.

Diseases and problems of the digestive system

Everybody has probably suffered from some sort of 'tummy trouble' at some time. These problems are not usually serious, and you recover within a few days. Constipation occurs if faeces do not move quickly enough through the large intestine. If they spend longer in the large intestine, more water is removed and the faeces are harder than usual. This causes difficulty and discomfort as they pass through the anus. Diarrhoea is the opposite of constipation. The faeces move too quickly through the large intestine. Not enough water is removed and the faeces leave the body in a semi-liquid state. Food poisoning may occur if there is something wrong with the food you have eaten. Both bacteria and viruses in food can cause food poisoning Bacteria in food can multiply if food is not kept under hygienic conditions. Some bacteria release harmful substances which can cause the stomach to feel upset and uncomfortable. Although this can be unpleasant, it is not usually dangerous. Food poisoning may, however, cause serious illness in small babies, elderly people, and people in poor health.

The appendix may get infected with germs. If the germs multiply, they can cause severe infection. This condition is called appendicitis. Doctors treat appendicitus by performing an operation in which they remove the appendix.

The contents of the stomach are strongly acidic. If the lining of the stomach is damaged by an infection or by medicines such as aspirin, the acid may penetrate and cause a painful area called an ulcer. People who have ulcers are treated with tablets which reduce the amount of acid produced.

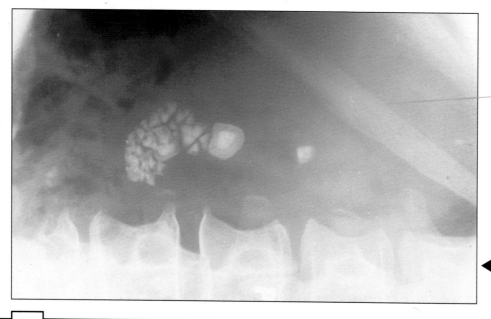

◀ **Doctors can detect gall stones by looking at an X-ray.**

Insulin helps to control the amount of glucose (sugar) in the blood. If the pancreas does not produce enough insulin, or if the body cannot use insulin properly, the amount of sugar in the blood cannot be controlled. If the level of sugar is too high, sugar will be excreted in the urine. If it gets very low, the brain will be unable to work properly and the person falls into a coma. This condition is called diabetes and people who suffer from it are called diabetics. Some diabetics control their diabetes by injecting insulin, while others manage their diabetes by following a strict diet.

Bile contains mineral salts and other substances, which are usually dissolved in the liquid bile. However, sometimes these salts solidify and harden, forming gall stones. If these stones block the bile duct, bile cannot leave the gall bladder. A person with gall stones may also suffer from jaundice. The skin and eyes become yellow because bile pigments (pigments are substances that give bile its strong green colour) get into the bloodstream. People who suffer from gall stones may have attacks of pain, especially after a fatty meal. They are advised to follow a fat-free diet, to avoid bile being produced to digest their food, and the stones will usually be removed by a surgeon.

Some diabetics can control their disease by daily injections of insulin.

The liver

The liver is a large, reddish-brown organ which lies on the right side of the upper **abdomen**, partly overlapping the stomach. It has two lobes. The right lobe is smaller than the left, and the gall bladder is tucked behind it. The liver is involved in hundreds of different chemical reactions, and controls and regulates many processes in the body. It is made up of tiny, six-sided units called lobules. Sheets of liver cells fan out from the centre of each lobule. Blood flows through the spaces between these sheets of cells.

Small branches of the **hepatic** artery and hepatic portal vein, which run between the lobules, bring blood from the heart and the intestine. A tiny vein runs up the centre of each lobule. These central veins join up with each other and eventually form the hepatic vein, carrying blood away from the liver and back to the heart. Tiny tubes called bile ducts run between the lobules, collecting bile. These carry bile to the gall bladder.

The liver has many different jobs to do:

It regulates the amount of sugar in the blood by taking out glucose and storing it as **glycogen**. When the blood sugar level begins to drop, the liver changes the glycogen back into glucose and releases it into the blood.

It breaks down unwanted amino acids and stores them as glycogen. The waste product of this break down is urea. This is carried away from the liver in the blood and is later removed by the kidneys.

It regulates the levels of **vitamins** and **minerals** in the blood by storing them until they are needed.

It removes iron from the haemoglobin of broken-down red blood cells, and stores it until it is needed to make new red blood cells.

It produces bile for digesting fats. Up to a litre of bile is produced every day. Bile contains bilirubin, which is made from broken-down haemoglobin.

It filters poisons, germs and drugs, making them harmless and keeping the body safe.

It makes fibrinogen (which is used in blood clotting) and other blood plasma proteins.

The chemical reactions that take place in the liver produce a lot of heat. This heat is circulated by the blood, and helps maintain body temperature.

The liver is a very large organ, and lies on the right side of the upper abdomen. ▶

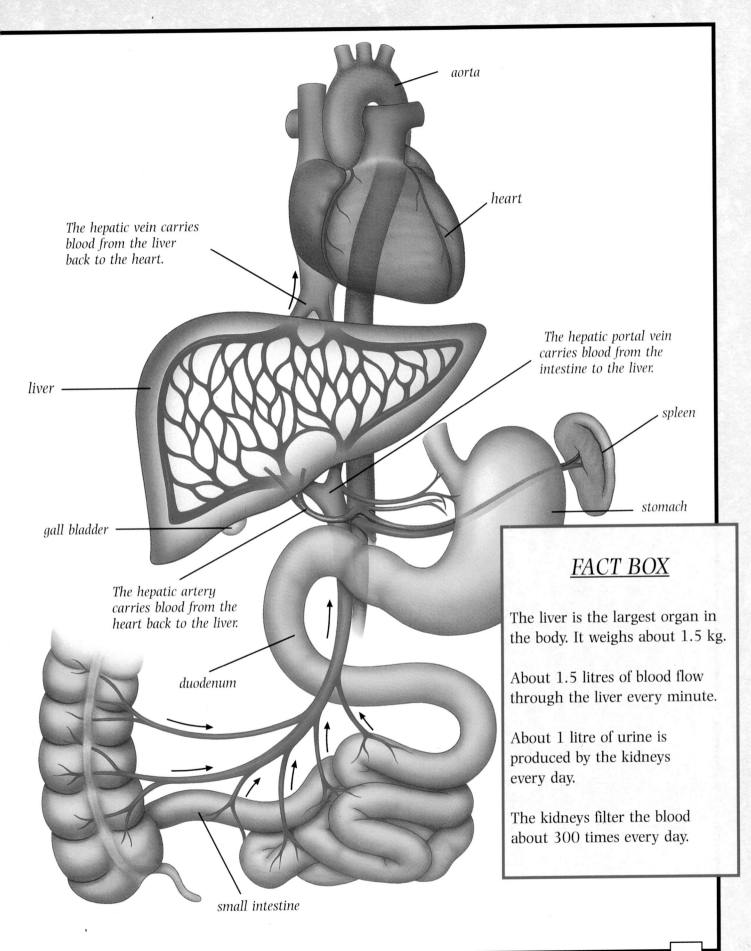

aorta

heart

The hepatic vein carries blood from the liver back to the heart.

The hepatic portal vein carries blood from the intestine to the liver.

spleen

liver

stomach

gall bladder

The hepatic artery carries blood from the heart back to the liver.

duodenum

small intestine

FACT BOX

The liver is the largest organ in the body. It weighs about 1.5 kg.

About 1.5 litres of blood flow through the liver every minute.

About 1 litre of urine is produced by the kidneys every day.

The kidneys filter the blood about 300 times every day.

The kidneys

We have two kidneys. Each is an oval shape, 10 cm long and 5 cm wide. They lie at the back of the body, just above the waist. The kidneys filter blood to:
control the levels of water and salts
get rid of urea, a waste product from the liver.

Blood travels to the kidneys via the **renal** artery. After the kidneys have filtered the blood, it is carried back to the heart via the renal vein.

There are three mains areas to each kidney. The outer layer is the cortex, the middle layer is the medulla, and in the centre is a space called the pelvis. Small branches of the renal artery carry blood to the cortex. Here, the blood enters a bunch of tiny tubules called a glomerulus. Each glomerulus sits inside a cup-shaped bag, called a nephron. As blood flows through the tubules, the liquid part of the blood filters through into the nephron. The substances in blood needed by the body move back into the bloodstream, leaving the waste materials behind in the nephron. The 'cleaned' blood travels back along capillaries until it eventually reaches the renal vein. It is then carried back to the heart. The waste materials left in the nephron flow down the tubules and into larger tubes called collecting ducts. The liquid is called urine. It leaves the kidney via a tube, the ureter, and is carried to the bladder. It is stored in the bladder until it can be released from the body when going to the toilet. Urine leaves the body via a narrow tube called the urethra. A ring of muscle opens and closes the exit of the urethra, and this muscle is usually under voluntary control.

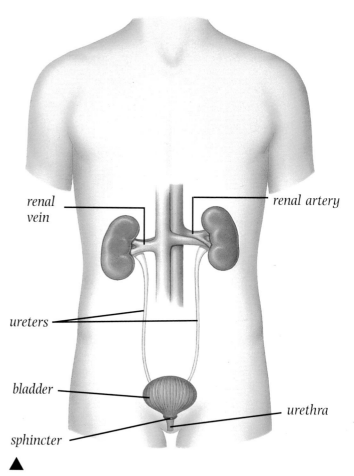

renal vein · renal artery · ureters · bladder · urethra · sphincter

▲

The kidneys lie at the back of the body, just above the waist.

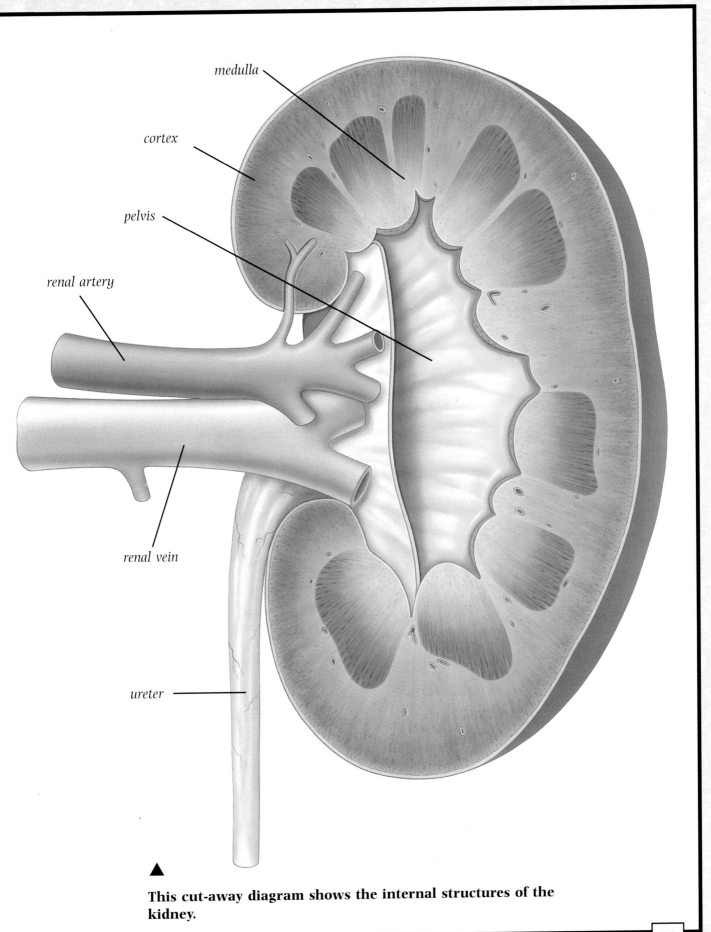

medulla

cortex

pelvis

renal artery

renal vein

ureter

▲
This cut-away diagram shows the internal structures of the kidney.

Diseases of the liver and kidneys

Several problems can affect the liver and kidneys. Some cannot be prevented, while others can. Alcohol can kill liver cells. Drinking large amounts of alcohol over a long period of time can damage the liver very badly. The tissue becomes fibrous and cannot carry out normal liver functions. This is called cirrhosis and can eventually lead to liver failure and death. Cirrhosis can also be caused by other factors, such as infection with hepatitis virus.

The skin and eyes of a person suffering from jaundice look yellow. This happens when too much bilirubin (the pigment found in bile) enters the blood. The main causes of jaundice are gall stones blocking the bile duct, and from hepatitis due to virus infections.

Mineral salts extracted from the blood in the kidneys are usually dissolved in liquid, but sometimes they solidify and form hard lumps called kidney stones. If they are very large, they may be removed by surgery. If they are small enough, they can often be treated by using a laser beam. This shatters them into tiny fragments which can then leave the kidneys in the urine.

Healthy liver cells can carry out liver functions efficiently.

Liver tissue that is damaged cannot function properly.

An 'artificial kidney' (dialysis machine) can filter a person's blood if their kidneys are unable to do so.

▼

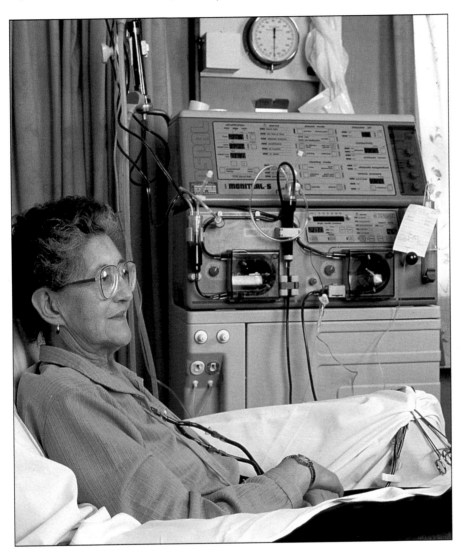

Kidney failure means that a person's kidneys have stopped working. This may be the result of an accident or disease. The body can function with just one kidney, but if both kidneys fail, blood cannot be cleaned and the person would die. Patients with kidney failure can clean their blood using an artificial kidney, or dialysis machine. The patient's blood is pumped into the machine, filtered, and then pumped back into their body. They may have to attach themselves to their kidney machine several times a week for two to four hours at a time An alternative to dialysis by a machine is a kidney transplant. The patient's diseased kidney is removed and replaced with a healthy one from a kidney donor.

◀ **Two sections of liver, one showing healthy liver cells and the other showing damaged liver cells.**

Types of food

The body uses food for energy, growth and repair, and to stay healthy. We need energy to make our muscles and organs work. To grow, our body needs to make new cells, and to stay heathy it needs to replace worn-out cells. The body can only do this by using nutrients from food. Without the right nutrients, the body would soon become diseased and unhealthy.

Different foods contain different nutrients. The body uses each nutrient for specific purposes. Food can be split into four main groups, depending on the nutrients they contain:

 1. Meat, fish, eggs, nuts and pulses, (lentils, chick-peas and beans) – these are rich in **proteins.**
 2. Fruit and vegetables – these are rich in vitamins and fibre.
 3. Dairy products – these are rich in fats and proteins.
 4. Bread, biscuits, cereals – these are rich in carbohydrates.

The body uses proteins for growth and repair, fats and carbohydrates for energy, and vitamins and minerals for general good health. Fibre is not actually digested and absorbed by the body, but it is very important in the diet. It makes digested food in the colon bulkier and helps it to retain water. The food can then move more easily and quickly through the colon, and the faeces are softer.

To stay healthy, the body needs a wide range of different nutrients – a balanced diet. To make sure the body gets the nutrients it needs, foods from each of the food groups need to be eaten every day.

FACT BOX

An average adult eats about 500 kg of food each year.

The energy in food is measured in kilojoules (kJ), after the famous British physicist, James Prescott Joule.

 If you take in more food than you use, the surplus is stored as fat.

Water is essential for life. About 75 per cent of the body is water. Humans can live for several weeks without food, but can only survive a few days without water.

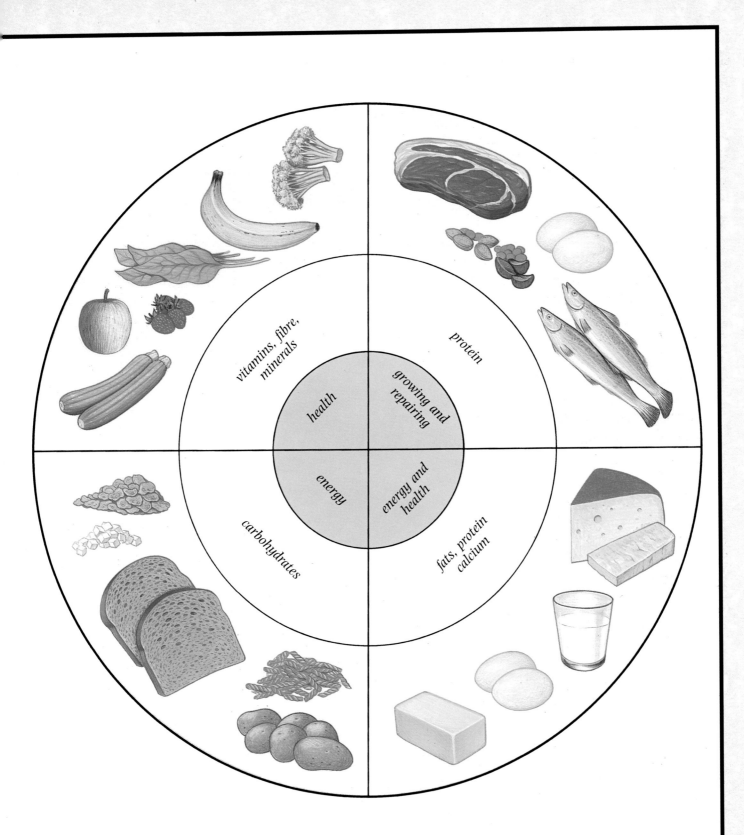

vitamins, fibre, minerals

protein

health

growing and repairing

energy

energy and health

carbohydrates

fats, protein calcium

Different types of food contain different nutrients. To make sure you eat a balanced diet, try to eat something from each of the sections of the food wheel every day.

Proteins

Proteins are used to make the main structural parts of the body. They are essential for the body to grow properly and to repair damaged and worn-out tissues. Proteins can also be used for energy, but this is not their most important function.

Doctors recommend that, every day, an average person needs about 0.57 g of protein for every kilogram of body mass. For example, a body mass of 35 kg will need to eat 35 x 0.57 (roughly 20 g) of protein. Proteins are found in meat, fish, eggs, dairy products, beans and pulses. Proteins are very long, complicated molecules, and are made up of smaller molecules called amino acids which are strung together like beads on a necklace. There are twenty different amino acids. The body cannot make amino acids, but it can change some amino acids into other amino acids. There are eight amino acids, called essential amino acids, which cannot be formed by the body. These essential amino acids have to be obtained from food. If the diet does not contain these amino acids, protein-deficiency diseases may develop.

Most animal proteins contain all the essential amino acids, but vegetarians have to make sure that they eat a range of different protein-rich foods. Few plants contain all the essential amino acids, but by including a mixture of cereals, beans and pulses in their diet, vegetarians can make sure that they do get all the essential amino acids needed by the body for growth and repair of tissues.

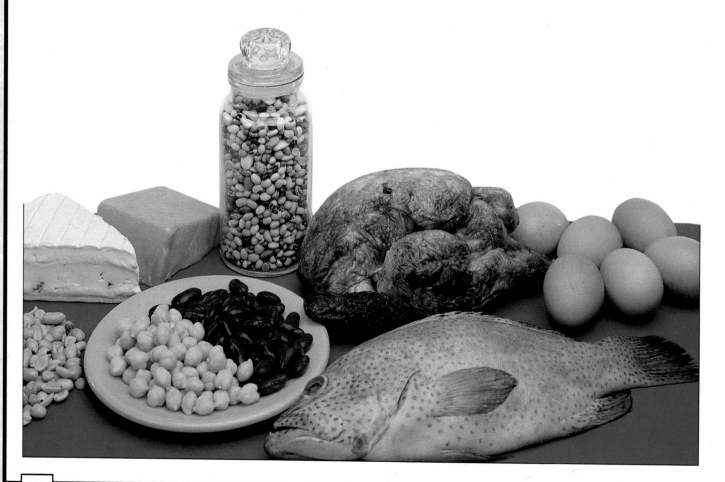

When proteins are digested, they are broken down into individual amino acids. The body can then use these as building blocks to create new proteins. These new proteins are used to build cells and tissues such as skin, bone and muscle. The body cannot store amino acids or proteins. If more are taken in than needed, the extra amino acids are taken to the liver. In the liver they are converted into glycogen (a type of sugar) which can be stored or used for energy.

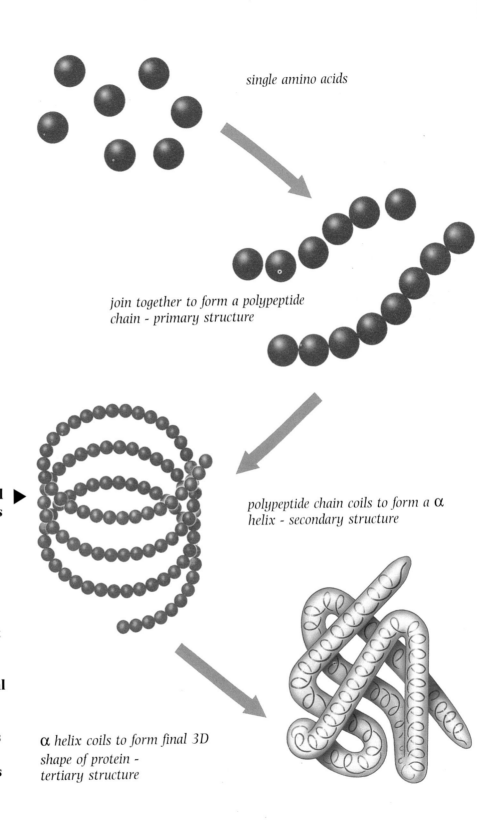

single amino acids

join together to form a polypeptide chain - primary structure

polypeptide chain coils to form a α helix - secondary structure

α helix coils to form final 3D shape of protein - tertiary structure

The arrangement of individual amino acids to form a chain is called the primary structure of a protein molecule. The individual amino acids can link together across the chain, making it loop round. These cross-links are called the secondary structure. Most proteins are held together by more links to form a complicated three-dimensional shape. Some proteins have more than one chain, and some contain other molecules too. The three-dimensional shape of a protein is called its tertiary structure.

◄ **Meat, fish, eggs and milk are all good sources of protein. Vegetarians can get the proteins they do not get in meat or fish from beans, pulses and cereals.**

Fats and carbohydrates

Fats and **carbohydrates** are used for energy. Fats are an excellent source of energy. Every gram of fat provides nearly 40 kj of energy. If more fats are eaten than required by the body, they can be stored under the skin in a layer of special cells (adipose cells). When the body needs energy, this fat store can be used. It also acts as insulation, trapping heat inside the body, which helps to keep it warm. Fats are found in animals and plants. Sources of animal fats are meat, dairy products and egg yolk. Plant fats are usually liquid at room temperature and are called oils. Many nuts and seeds contain oils, and are often used in cooking, for example, olive and sunflower oil.

Fats are long molecules made up of smaller molecules called fatty acids. There are many different types of fatty acid, which make many different types of fat. Scientists usually split fatty acids into two main groups, saturated and unsaturated fatty acids. Plant fats contain more unsaturated fatty acids than animal fats, and these are thought to be healthier.

The amount of energy needed by the body every day depends on age, gender and activity.
▼

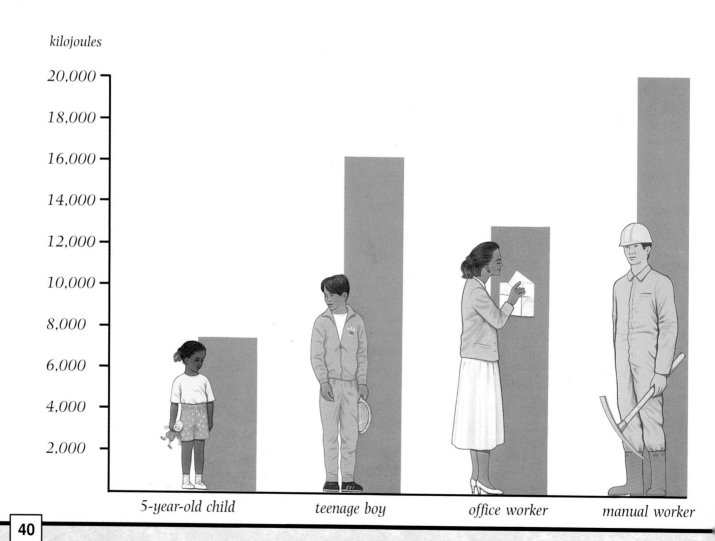

kilojoules

20,000
18,000
16,000
14,000
12,000
10,000
8,000
6,000
4,000
2,000

5-year-old child   teenage boy   office worker   manual worker

Carbohydrates are good sources of energy too, but they provide less than half as much energy as fats. One gram of carbohydrate gives about 16 kJ of energy. If more carbohydrate is taken in than the body needs, the surplus goes to the liver. In the liver, it is either converted into glycogen and stored in the muscles and liver, or it is converted into fats and stored under the skin.

Some foods, such as fruits, contain sugar naturally. Other foods, such as jam, cake, biscuits and sweets are manufactured and have sugar added to them. This added sugar is made from sugar beet and sugar cane. Different types of food contain different types of sugar. Starch is found in plant foods such as potatoes and rice.

Cereals like wheat contain a lot of starch and are often ground into flour, and used to make foods such as bread and pasta.

Different people use different amounts of energy, depending on their age, gender and daily activities. A five-year-old child will use nearly 8,000 kJ each day, but a man doing a heavy manual job will use about 20,000 kJ. An older woman may use only 11,000 kJ and an office worker 12,000 kJ.

Meat, dairy products, nuts and seeds are all rich in fats. Starchy foods (like bread, pasta and potatoes) and sweet foods (like cakes, biscuits and sweets) are all good sources of carbohydrate.

▼

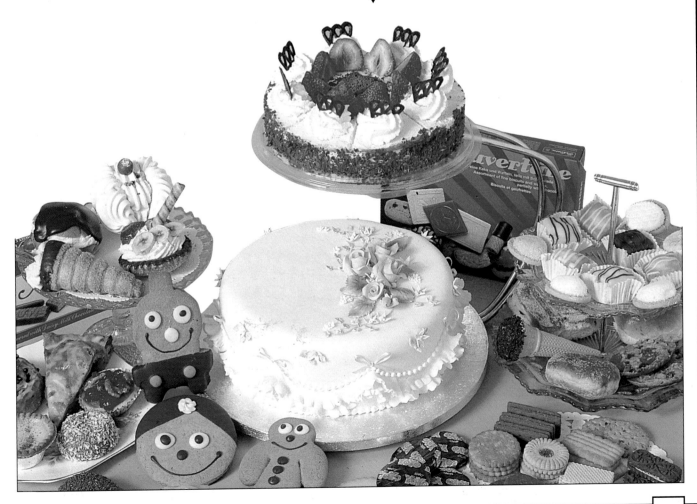

Vitamins and minerals

Vitamins are a special group of chemicals which are essential in very small amounts. They help to control the chemical reactions that take place inside the body cells. Each vitamin has its own special job to do, and if our diet is deficient in any of the vitamins we can become ill.

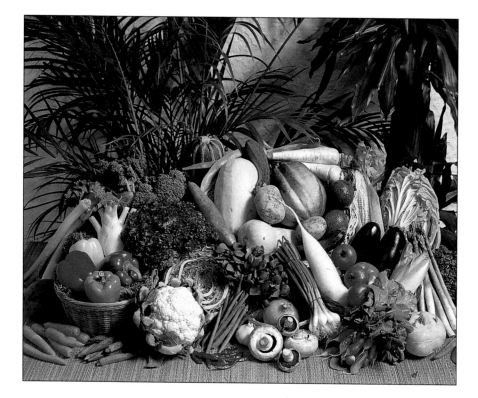

There are at least fifteen vitamins, named by letters. Our bodies cannot make vitamins, so we have to include vitamin-rich foods in our diet. Different types of food contain different vitamins. Vitamin A is found in fish oils, dairy products and liver. It is important for keeping the eyes healthy, and for being able to see in dim light. Several vitamins grouped together are called the B vitamins. These are found in whole cereals, peas and beans. They have a wide variety of functions and are important in maintaining good general health. Fresh fruit (especially oranges) and vegetables are excellent sources of vitamin C. This vitamin is important for the growth and maintenance of all parts of the body, and for healing wounds. It may also help protect against cancer in later life. Vitamin D is found

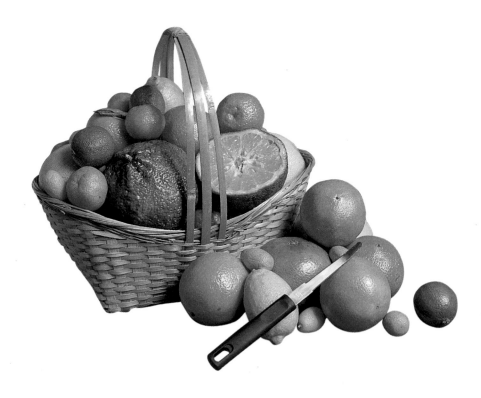

in dairy products, eggs, liver and fish oil. The body can also make vitamin D in the skin when it is exposed to sunlight. Without it, bones cannot form properly. They stay soft for too long, and the weight of the child makes them bend. In adults, lack of vitamin D can make the bones soft so they break easily. It is possible to have too much vitamin D, and this causes calcium to be deposited in other parts of the body, such as kidneys and lungs. Foods rich in vitamin E include milk, eggs and some green vegetables. It plays an important part in ensuring that reproductive organs stay healthy. Vitamin K is found in green vegetables such as spinach. Without it, blood cannot clot properly.

Although we can get all the vitamins we need by eating a balanced diet, some people like to ensure they get enough by taking vitamin tablets. Too much of some vitamins can be dangerous though, so it is important not to exceed the dose recommended on the bottle.

Minerals are needed in very small quantities. Each mineral contains chemical elements that are essential for our bodies to operate properly. Some minerals are needed as building blocks for growth and repair, while others are involved in controlling chemical reactions inside the body.

Calcium is essential for strong bones and teeth. It also helps blood to clot and is involved in making muscles contract.

Dairy products and fish are good sources of calcium. Sodium helps muscles to contract and helps pass messages along nerves. We get sodium from salt, either from the food itself or from extra salt that we put on the food before it is eaten. Salt is important in our diet, but too much can lead to high blood pressure. Iron is needed to make haemoglobin, a chemical in blood that carries oxygen around the body. Good sources of iron include liver, nuts and green vegetables. Without iron, blood cannot carry enough oxygen and anaemia develops. Symptoms of anaemia are tiredness and a pale skin. Iodine is an essential part of a hormone made by the thyroid gland in the neck. Iodine is found in fish oils and most vegetables. Lack of iodine may lead to goitre, a condition in which the thyroid gland swells.

A lack of iodine may lead to goitre in the neck.
▼

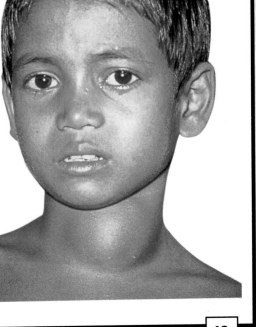

◀ **Fruit and vegetables are rich in vitamins. Cooking can destroy vitamins, so it is important to include some raw fruit and vegetables in your diet.**

Eating for health

To stay healthy, it is important to eat a balanced diet. The best way to do this is to try to make sure that you eat something from each of the main food groups each day.

It is important to get the balance right. If you eat more energy-rich foods than your body can use up, the extra energy will be stored as fat under your skin. Being very overweight is unhealthy because the heart has to work harder to pump blood around the body. It is just as important to eat enough energy-rich foods, otherwise your body will start to use up any stored fat to supply the energy it needs. Once it has used up fat, it will begin to use up muscle tissue too, and you can end up feeling very tired and weak. Losing too much weight can be very dangerous, because eventually, important organs such as the kidneys, heart and liver cannot function properly.

Water is an important part of everybody's diet. It is lost constantly from the body by sweating, breathing and urinating, and must be replaced by drinking regularly.

It makes sense to avoid foods that will damage your body. Some foods needed by the body are not good for the body in large quantities. Too much fat can cause a greasy skin and spots, and too many sugary foods and drinks can cause tooth decay.

Some manufactured foods have chemicals added to make them look more attractive and to change the flavours, but not all these additives are good for the body. Some ready-made foods have been through so many processes that, although they may taste good and be filling, they may have very little actual food value in them.

Drugs are chemicals that affect the mind and body. Medicines are drugs that are taken to cure illness. Provided the instructions are followed, medicines are not likely to damage health. Some people take drugs that have not been prescribed for them, because they enjoy the way they make them feel, but these effects do not last long. The damage drugs can do to the mind and body can last forever. All drugs can be dangerous, if used in the wrong way, and some lethal.

Many people enjoy drinking alcohol and doctors generally agree that small amounts of alcohol are unlikely to do permanent damage. But heavy drinking can have serious effects. Alcohol speeds up the destruction of brain cells, and the liver that processes the alcohol is eventually damaged by it. Alcohol also makes blood vessels get narrower, so the heart has to work very hard to pump blood through them. This puts the heart under a lot of strain, and the heart muscle becomes weak and enlarged.

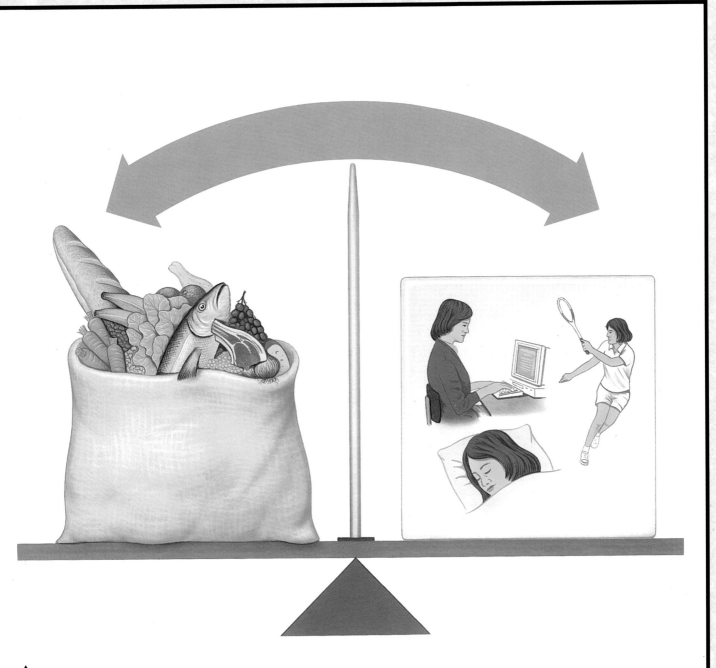

▲
Try to balance the amount of food you eat and the amount of activity you do.

Glossary

abdomen   part of the body containing the stomach, bowels and reproductive organs

amino acids   small molecules that are joined together to make proteins

bile   a liquid made by the liver which helps to break down fats

capillary   tiny, thin-walled blood vessel

carbohydrates   nutrients needed for energy

chyme   partly digested food that leaves the stomach

digestion   the process of breaking down food into small units which the body can use

enzymes   chemicals that break down large molecules into smaller ones

faeces   solid waste material that leaves the body

fats   nutrients needed for energy and energy storage

fatty acids   small molecules that are joined together to make fats

gastric   to do with the stomach

glucose   a type of sugar that the body can use for energy

glycogen   a type of sugar that the body can store

hepatic   to do with the liver

insulin   hormone involved in controlling the level of sugar in the bloodstream

lacteal   tiny, thin-walled tube carrying lymph

lymph   watery liquid that flows through the lymphatic system

minerals   chemicals in food that are needed, in very small amounts, for growth and repair

nutrients   parts of foods that are needed by the body to keep it in good working order

peristalsis   wave of muscular movement that pushes food through the digestive system

plaque   a layer of bacteria that can build up on the teeth

proteins   nutrients needed by the body for growth and repair

renal   to do with the kidneys

saliva   digestive juice made by salivary glands in the mouth

vitamins   chemicals in food that are needed in very small amounts for health

Books to Read

Digestion: Jenny Bryan (Wayland, 1992)

What's Inside Us?: Anita Ganeri (Macdonald Young Books, 1994)

Food and Digestion: Steve Parker (Watts Books, 1989)

The Human Body (Heinemann Library, 1994)

Index

Numbers in **bold** refer to illustrations